BEYOND TRAUMA CARE

BEYOND TRAUMA CARE

COMBINING THE SCIENCE OF
HEALING WITH THE
POWER OF RELATIONSHIPS

MATT OBERT, LCSW

ROOTED IN CHADDOCK'S MISSION
TO HEAL CHILDREN AND FAMILIES

Chaddock

BEYOND TRAUMA CARE
COMBINING THE SCIENCE OF HEALING WITH THE POWER OF RELATIONSHIPS
BY MATT OBERT, LCSW

The names and details of the people and situations described in this book have been changed or presented in composite form in order to ensure the privacy of those with whom the author and organization have served.

DTAP® is a registered trademark of Chaddock.

Published by

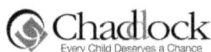 Chaddock
Every Child Deserves a Chance

www.chaddock.org

Cover design and interior layout by pearcreative.ca
Edited by coastalediting.com

ISBN: 979-8-9918469-2-9 (Print)
ISBN: 979-8-9918469-3-6 (eBook)

To every child who has ever been told they were "too much" or "not enough"—may you know that you are deeply seen, wholly loved, and capable of extraordinary healing.

To the parents, caregivers, teachers, clinicians, and leaders who choose connection over control and hope over fear—this book is for you.

In loving memory of Dr. Debbie Reed and Dwayne Charles "D.D." Fischer, whose vision and leadership shaped the heart of Chaddock and inspired this work.

And to my greatest sources of joy—my wife Amy and our children Jacob, Nathan, Emily, and Mathias—thank you for teaching me daily what it means to love deeply, lead with faith, and never lose hope.

ACKNOWLEDGMENTS

The Developmental Trauma and Attachment Program (DTAP®) represents years of learning, reflection, and growth at Chaddock. It is the result of collective dedication to providing hope and healing to children and families who need both.

We want to especially acknowledge the remarkable Chaddock employees—past and present—whose dedication, leadership, and creativity have shaped DTAP from its earliest beginnings to its continued success. Your commitment to healing, innovation, and excellence is at the heart of this work.

We also recognize that we have not made this journey alone. Thousands of volunteers, donors, community partners, and supporters have walked beside us over the years. Your generous contributions of time, resources, expertise, encouragement, and prayers have made the difference between being good and becoming truly great.

Your support has allowed us to grow, innovate, and deliver world-class care to some of the most vulnerable children and families in the nation.

To all who have shared in this mission of hope and healing, we offer our deepest gratitude. We could not have done this vital work without you.

CONTENTS

Acknowledgments   vii

Introduction   1

CHAPTER 1
Why the World Needs the Chaddock Way   5

CHAPTER 2
Foundations of Healing—Core Components of DTAP®   9

CHAPTER 3
Strategic Alignment—Leading with Purpose, People, Practice, and Progress   17

CHAPTER 4
Developing Your People and Culture   23

CHAPTER 5
From Information to Transformation—Training with Fidelity   29

CHAPTER 6
Making It Stick—Monitoring, Accountability, and Fidelity   37

CHAPTER 7
Scaling Up and Spreading Out   43

CHAPTER 8
Faith at the Center—Spiritual Leadership in a Secular World   51

CHAPTER 9
Systems Change in Action—Leading with the DTAP® Framework   57

CHAPTER 10
Case Studies and Stories from the Field   67

CHAPTER 11
The Strategic Playbook   73

CHAPTER 12
Conclusion—Becoming a Lighthouse of Hope   79

CHAPTER 13
Voices of Transformation—Testimonials from the DTAP® Journey   83

CHAPTER 14
Bringing DTAP® to Life—The Path to Certification and Fidelity   87

APPENDIX A
Quick-Start Leadership Action Checklist   93

APPENDIX B
Tools and Resources for Implementation   97

APPENDIX C
Frequently Asked Questions About DTAP®   105

References   109

About the Author   111

Chaddock

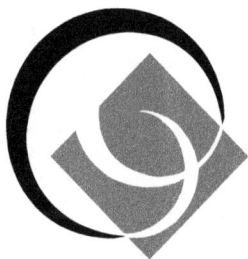

Every Child Deserves a Chance

INTRODUCTION

Welcome to *Beyond Trauma Care*—a blueprint for leaders and organizations who want to transform how they serve children and families impacted by trauma and disrupted attachment.

This book is for you if you are:
- A CEO or executive director of a nonprofit, faith-based agency, or child welfare organization seeking to create a culture of healing.
- A clinical director or therapist ready to move beyond techniques toward a relationship-centered, systems-wide model of care.
- An educator or school leader working to make trauma-informed and attachment-based practices more than slogans on the wall.
- A policy advocate or funder aiming to support sustainable, evidence-informed change.

Beyond Trauma Care introduces the Chaddock Way, rooted in our Developmental Trauma and Attachment Program (DTAP®)—a comprehensive, relationship-centered model of care developed through decades of practice and faith-informed leadership. DTAP is the combination of the science of healing with the power of relationships. DTAP is recognized on the California Evidence-Based Clearinghouse for Child Welfare (CEBC), affirming its structured and clearly defined approach to addressing complex trauma and attachment challenges in children and families.

The Chaddock Way is not about enforcing a single set of rules or claiming we have all the answers. Instead, it's about sharing what we've learned through decades of practice, research, and faith-informed leadership—offering a framework that others can adapt to their own communities and contexts. While the DTAP model itself is universal and adaptable, we share our "way" as an example of how these principles can be woven deeply into an organization's culture.

Too often, trauma-informed care becomes a checklist, a poster, or a single training that fails to transform culture. This guide is for leaders who want to do the real work of change.

You'll find not just knowledge but a framework for building organizations and systems that truly heal:

- Shaping policies and practices that reflect what we know about attachment and brain development
- Equipping teams with skills to create safety, connection, and long-term transformation
- Leading with courage, humility, and deep commitment to the power of relationships

If you are ready to ask hard questions, examine entrenched practices, and lead from a place of compassion and conviction, welcome. You're in the right place.

CHAPTER 1

WHY THE WORLD NEEDS THE CHADDOCK WAY

Over the past two decades, interest in trauma-informed care has surged. Across the country, organizations have adapted the language of being "trauma-informed," displaying posters on walls and hosting one-time trainings.

Yet despite good intentions, too many systems stop short of true transformation. Trauma-informed care has become a buzzword, often stripped of its power to drive meaningful change. Because true healing requires more than knowledge. It demands a new way of seeing, leading, and relating.

This is where we introduce the Chaddock Way.

The Chaddock Way and DTAP®

Developed over decades of practice, clinical expertise, and reflective leadership, the Chaddock Way represents more than just another trauma framework. It is our way of integrating the Developmental Trauma and Attachment Program (DTAP)—a comprehensive, evidence-informed model grounded in developmental psychology, attachment science, and our agency's faith-informed values. Together with the organizational culture, leadership practices, and relational commitments that bring it to life, the Chaddock Way makes healing both real and sustainable.

We share it not as the only way but as one example of how these principles can be lived out in daily practice. Our hope is that you will adapt what resonates, challenge what doesn't, and make it your own in the service of healing children, families, staff, and communities.

Integrating Relationship, Regulation, and Competence

DTAP itself is different because it integrates what so many systems treat separately: emotional regulation, neurobiological development, safe environments, secure relationships, and long-term transformation. It speaks to the core of human development, honoring a simple truth: Healing happens in the context of relationships. Not just any relationships, but intentional, attuned, and enduring ones.

Too often, systems designed to care for children become systems of control. The behaviors of traumatized children—defiance, withdrawal, aggression, disconnection—are treated as problems to manage, rather than signals to understand. Staff may receive training in techniques, but their mindsets remain unchanged. Leaders may focus on compliance instead of connection. Policies may be trauma-aware in writing, yet the daily experiences of children in care tell a different story.

The Chaddock Way challenges this cycle.

Leadership for True Transformation

It offers more than awareness. It provides a road map for healing. It insists that systems built around fear, rigidity, or burnout can be transformed into communities rooted in safety, connection, and growth. But it starts with leadership—leaders willing to ask hard questions, examine their own practices, and lead with courage and compassion.

This book is for those leaders. For those who feel the weight of unmet needs and know that more policies or trainings alone won't fix what's broken.

For those who want to build organizations where children can truly heal—and where staff can thrive, not just survive.

For those willing to go beyond trauma care.

In the pages ahead, you will learn the foundations of DTAP, the strategic frameworks that align your mission with your methods, and the tools Chaddock uses to train, certify, and support healing-focused teams.

But first, we begin with a critical question, one every leader must ask: Are we creating systems that reflect what we know about healing, or are we perpetuating the very dynamics that retraumatize?

CHAPTER 2

FOUNDATIONS OF HEALING— CORE COMPONENTS OF DTAP®

Effective healing requires a clear, intentional path forward. Chaddock's Developmental Trauma and Attachment Program (DTAP) offers that path through a simple yet profound framework that guides clinical practice and shapes organizational culture: the DTAP Pyramid.

This pyramid is not just a clinical model; it is a leadership framework. It describes three interdependent phases, each building a secure foundation for the next, to support healing, personal development, and resilience.

The DTAP Pyramid Framework

The DTAP Pyramid reflects what we know from developmental psychology, attachment science, and brain-based research.

It follows a progression from safety (meeting survival needs), to connection and regulation (developing relational and emotional skills), and finally to reasoning and competence (higher-level problem-solving, mastery, and agency).

This hierarchy aligns with brain development:
- Lower brain functions focus on safety and survival.
- Midbrain systems support connection and emotional regulation.
- Higher cortical functions enable reasoning, planning, and competence.

DTAP recognizes that these phases are interdependent. Healing is not linear but layered, requiring us to reliably meet foundational needs before expecting advanced skills to develop.

DTAP's impact is supported by its listing on the California Evidence-Based Clearinghouse for Child Welfare (CEBC), where it is recognized as a structured, evidence-informed intervention for use with children and families impacted by trauma and disrupted attachment.

Safety

At the base of the DTAP Pyramid lies *safety*. Without this foundation, healing cannot begin.

Safety means more than the absence of physical danger. It includes emotional, relational, and cultural safety—a sense that children are protected, valued, and understood.

Safety requires:
- Clear expectations and dependable adults.
- Predictable routines and environments that feel calm and welcoming.
- Staff who demonstrate consistency, emotional availability, and attuned presence.

Organizations committed to DTAP must deliberately build safety into every layer of their work—from leadership decisions to staff-client interactions, from policy writing to daily greetings.

Without safety, the brain remains in a state of survival, and true growth cannot occur.

Connection and Regulation

Once safety is reliably in place, children can begin to develop *connection* and *regulation*.

Connection is the relational bridge that makes healing possible. Through safe, attuned relationships, children learn to trust again, take healthy risks, and experience co-regulation with caring adults. DTAP emphasizes that healing is not something done *to* someone, but something created *with* them.

Connection requires:
- Attuned, empathetic engagement from adults.
- Consistent, safe, relational presence, even during challenging moments.
- Culturally responsive practices that honor each child's identity and experience.

Regulation is the ability to manage emotions and behaviors. DTAP frames it as a developmental skill that must be taught and practiced. Dysregulation is not a moral failing or sign of defiance.

Staff learn to understand the neuroscience of dysregulation and model healthy coping strategies, helping children transition from reactive states into calm, engaged interactions that foster growth.

Supporting regulation means:
- Responding to emotional expression with understanding rather than punishment.
- Recognizing signs of stress in both children and staff.
- Practicing co-regulation consistently through calm, connected presence.

Connection and regulation provide the emotional stability necessary for learning, healthy relationships, and long-term healing.

Reasoning and Competence

As children experience safety, build connection, and develop regulation skills, they become ready to achieve *reasoning* and *competence*.

Reasoning refers to the child's growing capacity for problem-solving, perspective-taking, and self-reflection. It emerges only when lower brain systems are calmed and relational safety is established.

Competence goes beyond simple compliance or behavior management. It is about helping children recognize their strengths, develop new skills, and experience authentic success in relationships, academics, and self-expression.

DTAP-based organizations create opportunities for youth to:
- Achieve mastery and make meaningful contributions.
- Build a sense of agency and positive self-perception.
- Experience success that transforms their self-image from "I am broken" to "I am able."

Building reasoning and competence isn't an afterthought; it is an essential part of healing. It gives children the tools they need to navigate challenges and thrive beyond the walls of care.

Faith as a Guiding Value

While faith is not a formal component of the DTAP Pyramid, it is a guiding value that shapes Chaddock's approach.

Our faith heritage calls us to see the inherent worth of every child and family, to lead with compassion, humility, and hope— even when healing feels impossible.

Faith informs the way we approach our work, not by imposing beliefs but by recognizing that healing is meaningful, even sacred work. It reminds us that transformation is possible, even for wounds that seem beyond repair.

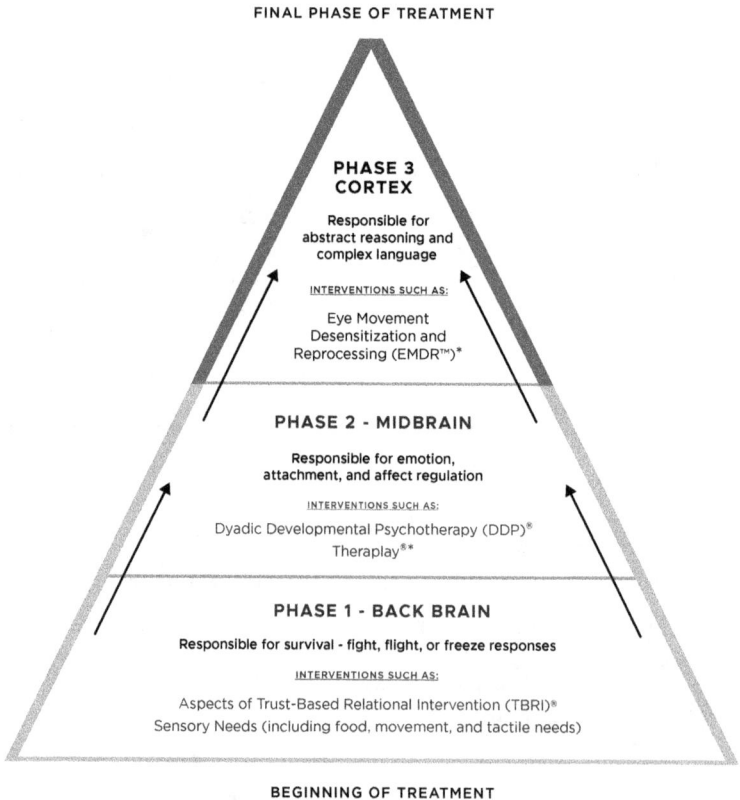

FINAL PHASE OF TREATMENT

PHASE 3 CORTEX

Responsible for abstract reasoning and complex language

INTERVENTIONS SUCH AS:

Eye Movement Desensitization and Reprocessing (EMDR™)*

PHASE 2 - MIDBRAIN

Responsible for emotion, attachment, and affect regulation

INTERVENTIONS SUCH AS:

Dyadic Developmental Psychotherapy (DDP)®
Theraplay®*

PHASE 1 - BACK BRAIN

Responsible for survival - fight, flight, or freeze responses

INTERVENTIONS SUCH AS:

Aspects of Trust-Based Relational Intervention (TBRI)®
Sensory Needs (including food, movement, and tactile needs)

BEGINNING OF TREATMENT

*Specific components of these models apply to lower levels of the pyramid as well.

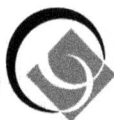

REFLECTION QUESTIONS

As you consider this framework, pause and reflect:

- Does your organization reliably establish safety at every level before supporting connection and regulation?
- Do your teams prioritize authentic relationships and attuned connection over compliance?
- Are staff trained and supported to model emotional regulation?
- Are children given opportunities to build reasoning and competence?
- Is your work grounded in purpose, meaning, and shared values?

The DTAP Pyramid is more than a clinical tool. It is a leadership framework. When it becomes the foundation of your organization's culture, you will see transformation not only in the lives of those you serve but also in the way your people serve them.

CHAPTER 3

STRATEGIC ALIGNMENT—LEADING WITH PURPOSE, PEOPLE, PRACTICE, AND PROGRESS

If the Developmental Trauma and Attachment Program is the blueprint for healing, then *strategic alignment* is the architectural integrity that holds the entire structure together.

Without clear goals, integrated systems, and intentional leadership, even the most promising models can fall short. Strategic alignment ensures that every layer of your organization—its people, processes, practices, and purpose—works in harmony to fulfill your mission.

At Chaddock, we don't believe in mission statements that hang on the wall and collect dust. We believe in a mission that breathes life into every decision—from budgeting and hiring to supervision and client care. This kind of alignment doesn't happen by accident. It is intentional. And it starts with strategy.

> **Chaddock's mission is to strengthen children and families through innovative trauma and attachment-based services.**

A strong strategic plan creates *clarity*. It empowers every team member to understand where the organization is going and how their role contributes to that journey. Strategic alignment isn't about rigid control; it's about ensuring that everyone is rowing in the same direction.

The Three-Year Strategic Framework

To help organizations achieve this, Chaddock uses a three-year strategic framework built on four essential pillars:

1. **Purpose**: What are we uniquely positioned to do?
2. **People**: How do we build a culture that attracts, develops, and retains mission-aligned team members?
3. **Practice**: How do we ensure that our daily actions, interventions, and decisions consistently reflect our values, mission, and model fidelity? Practice is the bridge between vision and action—it is where strategy becomes lived reality. It's about aligning routines, behaviors, and standards so that the mission isn't just spoken but embodied in every interaction.

4. **Progress:** How do we track what matters and ensure accountability?

Jim Collins's Hedgehog Concept[1]

This framework is strengthened by proven tools and concepts that help leaders focus their strategy on what matters most.

Jim Collins's Hedgehog Concept guides organizations in answering three critical questions:

1. What are we deeply passionate about?
2. What can we be the best in the world at?
3. What drives our resource engine?

These questions help leaders clarify their unique value, focus their efforts, and avoid mission drift.

Patrick Lencioni's Organizational Health[2]

We also draw on Patrick Lencioni's emphasis on organizational health. It's not enough to be "smart" or have good technical strategies; organizations must also be healthy.

Healthy organizations reduce confusion, improve morale and productivity, and retain their most talented people. This commitment to health is vital in trauma-informed systems,

---

1 Jim Collins, *Good to Great: Why Some Companies Make the Leap... and Others Don't* (New York: HarperBusiness, 2001), 95–96.

2 Patrick M. Lencioni, *The Advantage: Why Organizational Health Trumps Everything Else in Business* (San Francisco: Jossey-Bass, 2012), 5–7.

where staff well-being has a direct impact on the safety and healing of those they serve.

Chaddock's Strategic Planning Process

Every strategic planning process at Chaddock includes:
- Stakeholder listening sessions to understand needs and perspectives.
- SOAR assessments (Strengths, Opportunities, Aspirations, Results) to identify what's working and where to grow.
- Vision, mission, and values refreshers to ensure alignment with current realities and aspirations.
- A two-day planning retreat with cross-functional leadership teams to foster collaboration and clarity.
- Defined outcomes and measurable action steps to turn vision into reality.

When done well, strategic planning is not just a task on a checklist. It is a transformational experience.

It revitalizes staff.
It recenters the mission.
It brings clarity to chaos.
It aligns people, policies, and practices in service of healing.

Having established the pillars of Purpose and People, the chapters ahead will explore Practice and Progress—how our values take shape through action and lead to measurable growth.

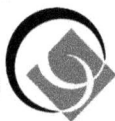

REFLECTION QUESTIONS

As you consider your own organization's strategy, take a
moment to reflect:

- Does your current strategy reflect
  your deepest values?
- Are your leaders aligned and empowered to act
  with clarity and confidence?
- Can every staff member see how their daily work
  contributes to your mission?

When strategy and healing go hand in hand,
organizations become unstoppable forces for good. That
is the power of alignment.

CHAPTER 4

DEVELOPING YOUR PEOPLE AND CULTURE

Culture isn't created in a workshop or captured in a manual. It is lived out in the small, daily interactions between people. It shows up in how staff speak to one another during stressful moments, how supervisors respond to mistakes, and how leaders model integrity, humility, and care.

At Chaddock, we believe that developing a trauma-responsive, attachment-informed organization begins with the intentional development of its people.

This chapter is about embedding the Developmental Trauma and Attachment Program's (DTAP's®) core values—safety, connection and regulation, and reasoning and competence— into your hiring, onboarding, supervision, and leadership practices. It's about building a culture that doesn't just tolerate people but forms them—shaping who they become and how they lead.

Start with Who—Hiring with Purpose

The best strategy in the world will fail without the right people. Culture-building starts with *who* you hire.

At Chaddock, we hire for heart first, skills second. We look for people who are curious, humble, mission-aligned, and resilient. Many can be trained in technique; fewer are prepared to enter into the sacred, complex, and meaningful work of healing relationships.

During interviews, we ask behavioral questions rooted in our values:

- How do you handle failure?
- How do you respond to someone in distress?
- What does accountability look like to you?

This allows us to see not just what candidates know but *who they are becoming.*

Orientation as Formation

Onboarding should be more than a checklist. It should be a *formation experience*—introducing employees not just to policies and procedures, but to the heart of your mission.

At Chaddock, new hires learn about the DTAP Pyramid, our organizational history, and the *why* behind our approach. We invite them into a story, not just a job.

We assign mentors to new employees, provide early opportunities for reflective supervision, and offer practical tools for managing dysregulation in both clients and themselves.

Onboarding is where values come alive. It's where expectations around culture are first modeled, and where new team members begin to feel that they belong.

Supervision as a Relationship

Supervision is often misunderstood as a compliance mechanism. At Chaddock, we see supervision as a relationship that mirrors the attachment dynamics we hope our staff will replicate with those they serve.

Supervision is about co-regulation, reflective listening, and growth-oriented feedback.

We train supervisors to be present, curious, and grounded. A simple but powerful question we use regularly is: "What do you need to feel safe and successful in your role this week?"

This reframes support as a partnership, not a transaction.

Coaching and Accountability

Culture is sustained not only through support but through accountability.

A strong DTAP-aligned culture doesn't mean permissiveness or avoidance. It means clearly naming what is expected—and supporting staff in meeting those expectations.

When someone acts outside of the model—perhaps by responding harshly to a child or disengaging from their team—we address it promptly and relationally. The goal is *learning, not punishment.*

Leaders are trained to deliver corrective feedback that is anchored in shared values, hope, and a commitment to growth.

Rituals, Recognition, and Renewal

Great cultures include rhythms that reinforce who you are and what you value.

At Chaddock, we intentionally build in practices to reflect, celebrate, and grow together:
- Staff shout-outs linked to our values
- Moments of silence or prayer at meetings (offered respectfully and inclusively)
- Ongoing DTAP training for all staff, not just clinicians
- Opportunities to attend retreats or conferences
- Celebrations that honor progress, resilience, and service

We also prioritize staff well-being through time off, flexibility, and access to mental health resources.

If we want our people to model *connection and regulation*, we must support them in living it.

Culture by Design, Not Default

Left unchecked, culture will evolve by default—and often not in a healthy direction.

A DTAP-aligned culture requires *intentional shaping*. Leaders must act as culture architects:
- Modeling the behaviors they want to see
- Rewarding what matters most
- Rooting every decision in the shared belief that relationships heal

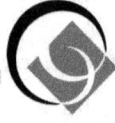

REFLECTION QUESTIONS

Here are questions we ask ourselves regularly—and invite you to consider:

- Does our culture reflect our stated values?
- Are our hiring and supervision practices aligned with DTAP principles?
- Do our rituals reinforce connection, reflection, and celebration?
- Are we forming people, or simply managing them?

A healthy, values-driven culture is the most sustainable intervention you can offer.

It's what keeps great staff.
It's what supports great outcomes.
It's what honors the meaningful, sacred work of healing.

And it begins with how you treat your people.

CHAPTER 5

FROM INFORMATION TO TRANSFORMATION— TRAINING WITH FIDELITY

A training program alone will not transform an organization. What truly matters is how deeply the knowledge is understood, practiced, implemented, and sustained over time.

Developmental Trauma and Attachment Program (DTAP®) training isn't simply an introduction to a model. It's an intentional process of reshaping how staff relate, respond, and reflect.

In this chapter, we'll explore how to move from information overload to genuine transformation through a structured, relational, and fidelity-driven approach to training.

A Culture of Ongoing Learning

At Chaddock, training is never a one-time event. It is woven into the fabric of our operations—a continual process that supports staff growth and organizational alignment.

From initial onboarding to quarterly workshops, consultation groups, and fidelity coaching, we emphasize lifelong learning. We believe people grow best in community, when supported by a culture that values humility, feedback, and shared growth.

Every DTAP-aligned training begins with a shared mindset: We are all learners. Whether someone is new direct care staff, an experienced therapist, or a senior leader, training is an opportunity to deepen relationships, improve practice, and strengthen alignment with our mission.

Foundational Training

All staff, regardless of role, begin their DTAP journey with foundational training. This includes:
- An introduction to trauma, attachment, and neurodevelopmental science.
- A detailed breakdown of the DTAP Pyramid: Safety, Connection and Regulation, and Reasoning and Competence.
- Real-life examples and video scenarios to make concepts real and practical.
- Interactive exercises to surface biases, assumptions, and challenges.

- Group dialogue and self-reflection.

The tone of this training is *relational and experiential.* We don't lecture; we engage. We invite *vulnerability, curiosity,* and *connection* so staff can see not only what they do, but *why* they do it.

Equipping DTAP-Certified Ambassadors and Coaches

One of the most powerful decisions an organization can make is to build internal capacity to support and sustain DTAP implementation over time.

Chaddock's DTAP Certification Program prepares staff to serve as DTAP-Certified Ambassadors and Coaches within their organization. Rather than delivering formal training sessions independently, these certified staff play a crucial role in maintaining fidelity, supporting colleagues, and modeling DTAP principles in daily work.

The certification process includes:
- A multi-day intensive learning experience.
- Mentorship and reflective supervision components.
- Practical demonstration of DTAP knowledge and application.
- Ongoing access to updated materials and consultation.

DTAP-Certified Ambassadors help ensure that new staff are oriented to DTAP values, offer informal refreshers, and provide in-the-moment coaching and support. They serve as internal champions for fidelity, helping embed DTAP practices into the culture of the organization.

DTAP Coaches and Ambassadors Defined

DTAP Coaches are experienced practitioners who model relational attunement, guide reflective practice, and use fidelity tools to help their teams translate DTAP theory into consistent, real-world action. They serve as mentors, providing feedback, support, and encouragement as staff deepen their skills and confidence.

DTAP Ambassadors are organizational leaders and culture carriers who embody the Chaddock Way and champion the integration of DTAP across all settings. They advocate for alignment among people, policy, and practice, ensuring the model's principles influence every layer of the organization. Together, Coaches and Ambassadors create a sustainable infrastructure that keeps DTAP alive in both heart and habit.

Note: A dedicated training program—designed to prepare staff to independently deliver the full DTAP training curriculum in the way master trainers do—is a separate, advanced level of preparation that can be developed in partnership with Chaddock.

Fidelity Monitoring

Training without fidelity is just performance. Fidelity ensures the model is delivered as intended.

We use structured fidelity tools to assess:

- The language and tone used by staff.
- Staff responsiveness to regulation needs.
- Alignment of daily practices with DTAP principles.
- The use of reflection and co-regulation in interactions.

Fidelity isn't about policing. It's about learning.

It provides leaders and teams with a shared language to discuss what's working, where support is needed, and how to grow together. It turns supervision into coaching. It transforms compliance checks into opportunities for connection and learning.

Tailoring for Role and Context

While DTAP is grounded in universal principles, its application must be adapted for role and context.

Chaddock provides role-specific training extensions for:
- Direct-care professionals.
- Therapists and clinicians.
- Educational staff and teachers.
- Supervisors and managers.
- Support and administrative roles.

We also tailor training by setting—whether it's residential, outpatient, school-based, or community programming. The principles remain constant, but the practices flex to fit real-world environments.

Creating Reflective Spaces

One of the most transformative elements of DTAP training is the use of *reflective spaces.*

These are structured opportunities for staff to process their work, receive feedback, and develop self-awareness. Consultation groups are facilitated by trained leaders who know how to hold space, ask powerful questions, and guide participants toward deeper insight.

Examples of reflection prompts include:
- "Where did you see safety and connection succeed this week?"
- "When did you struggle to regulate, and what was happening beneath the surface?"
- "What's one way that purpose or values showed up in your work this week?"

These sessions build team cohesion, reduce burnout, and strengthen fidelity.

From Training to Transformation

Ultimately, DTAP training isn't about delivering content. It's about creating cultural transformation.

That transformation happens when:
- Training is ongoing, role-specific, and reflective.
- Fidelity tools are used to measure and grow.
- Internal trainers are equipped and empowered.

- Reflection is prioritized over performance.

Training is only the beginning.

The true transformation comes when the principles of DTAP are no longer just taught, but *lived.*

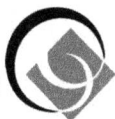

REFLECTION QUESTIONS

As you consider your own training approach, reflect on:
- Is training in your organization a one-time event or an ongoing journey?
- How do you ensure that training is relational, experiential, and engaging?
- How do you monitor fidelity without creating fear or defensiveness?
- Do your staff have opportunities to reflect, grow, and deepen their practice together?
- How might you build internal capacity to sustain this work over time?

When organizations commit to training with fidelity, they build cultures where healing is possible—not just for those they serve, but for the staff themselves.

CHAPTER 6

MAKING IT STICK—MONITORING, ACCOUNTABILITY, AND FIDELITY

Great models rarely fail because they're wrong; they fail because they aren't implemented with consistency. The Developmental Trauma and Attachment Program (DTAP®) is no exception.

Even the most well-intentioned organizations can drift off course without intentional structures for monitoring, coaching, and shared accountability.

This chapter equips you with the mindset and tools to ensure DTAP doesn't just get launched; it gets lived.

Fidelity as a Living Practice

Fidelity means practicing what you preach. It ensures that the core of DTAP—Safety, Connection and Regulation, and Reasoning and Competence—aren't just ideas but daily realities in your organization's interactions, practices, and culture.

At Chaddock, we've learned that fidelity is not a checkbox or an annual audit. It's a culture. A way of being. A shared commitment to integrity and alignment with our mission and values.

Defining Observable Behaviors

Fidelity checks can feel vague or even punitive if they're not clearly defined. That's why we break it down into *observable, specific behaviors* aligned with the DTAP:

- **Safety:** Does the environment feel predictable, calm, and respectful? Are relationships prioritized in interactions?
- **Connection and Regulation:** Are adults modeling self-regulation? Are children supported before being redirected?
- **Reasoning and Competence:** Are youth encouraged to try, fail, and succeed in developmentally appropriate tasks?

Beyond the pyramid, we also consider our organizational values like faith, relationships, responsibility, learning, and caring. These guide the overall tone of decisions, language, and care.

Each area has its own fidelity indicators that can be observed, measured, and coached in daily work.

Observational Tools and Walk-Throughs

At Chaddock, we use structured walk-throughs led by trained fidelity monitors.

These aren't designed to catch mistakes; they're designed to support *alignment and growth*. Observers spend time in classrooms, cottages, clinical settings, and even staff meetings.

They use a simple three-part feedback format:
1. **Affirmations**—What's going well and why it matters
2. **Curiosities**—Questions about intent or decision-making
3. **Opportunities**—Suggestions for deeper fidelity

Staff are encouraged to actively participate in these conversations. This approach builds trust, mutual learning, and a culture of continuous improvement.

Embedding Accountability at Every Stage

Fidelity doesn't belong to any one person or role; it's the responsibility of the whole system.

At Chaddock, accountability is layered throughout the organization:
- Frontline Staff: Receive regular coaching and supervision aligned with DTAP

- Mid-Level Leaders: Conduct peer walk-throughs and reinforce the culture through their own modeling
- Executive Leaders: Review fidelity reports, champion values, and build systems of support and sustainability

We don't separate performance from purpose. Accountability isn't about checking boxes. It's about ensuring that the way we do our jobs reflects why we do them.

Corrective Action that Builds, Not Breaks

When fidelity slips, how we respond matters deeply.

DTAP-aligned organizations address misalignment not with punishment, but with *clarity* and *care*. Corrective strategies might include:

- Additional coaching sessions.
- Restorative conversations to rebuild trust and understanding.
- Peer modeling or shadowing to demonstrate best practices.
- Realignment meetings with leadership to clarify expectations and values.

The goal is always *restoration, not removal.*

That said, persistent disregard for DTAP principles—even subtle forms of resistance—cannot be ignored. Children's healing depends on adult fidelity.

Using Data to Drive Growth

Fidelity tools should be simple enough to use regularly, yet rich enough to generate meaningful data.

At Chaddock, we collect and review:
- Observation trends over time.
- Training participation and completion rates.
- Notes from reflective supervision sessions.
- Staff and youth feedback surveys.

We analyze these data quarterly, identify gaps, and use the insights to inform strategic decisions.

Monitoring isn't separate from strategy; it is strategy in action.

Protecting What Matters Most

DTAP is powerful because it is relational. But that also means it is fragile. Left unchecked, stress, turnover, and competing demands can pull an organization away from its values.

That's why *fidelity is sacred*. It serves as the collective memory of who we are, why we do this work, and how we show up for children every day.

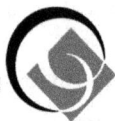

REFLECTION QUESTIONS

Before you move on to growth and expansion, pause to ask:
- Are we living what we say we believe?
- Are our systems reinforcing our values, or quietly eroding them?
- Do our staff feel safe, seen, and supported in staying aligned?
- How do we respond when practice drifts from our shared commitments?

Fidelity is not a burden. It's a gift.

It ensures the healing we offer is consistent, deep, and worthy of the children and families we serve.

CHAPTER 7

SCALING UP AND SPREADING OUT

If the Developmental Trauma and Attachment Program (DTAP®) can work in one setting, can it work in others?

Yes, but only with intention, adaptation, and unwavering commitment to fidelity.

While DTAP was born within Chaddock's residential treatment center, it was never meant to stay there. The principles of healing through Safety, Connection and Regulation, and Reasoning and Competence are relevant wherever children live, learn, play, or receive care.

This chapter examines how to scale DTAP across diverse settings—such as schools, outpatient clinics, and home-based services—and how to maintain its core principles.

It also addresses system-level advocacy and policy change, because healing at scale requires more than replication. It requires influence.

Beyond Residential Care

Residential settings provide high structure and consistency—ideal conditions for introducing and refining DTAP.

But many children will never enter residential care. And those who do must eventually return to homes, schools, and communities. Healing must go where they go.

Chaddock has successfully extended DTAP into:

- **Outpatient Therapy Services**: DTAP provides a framework for intake, treatment planning, and session delivery that focuses on building safety and co-regulation with families in their natural environments.
- **School Partnerships**: DTAP-aligned school environments emphasize relational discipline, classroom co-regulation strategies, staff attunement, and trauma-aware learning spaces.
- **Home-Based and Community Programs**: Family coaches and therapists trained in DTAP support biological, foster, or adoptive families as they navigate behavioral and relational challenges.

- **Foster Care Services**: DTAP principles guide foster care agencies in preparing, training, and supporting foster parents to create safe, attuned, and regulated homes. Emphasis is placed on understanding trauma responses, building secure relationships, and partnering with birth families and systems for long-term healing.

Each adaptation requires thoughtful training, clear expectations, and flexible implementation.

Training Systems, Not Just People

Scaling DTAP isn't just about training individuals. It's about introducing it to entire systems.

That means understanding the pressures, rhythms, and barriers unique to each context.

For example:
- In schools, time is segmented, roles are specialized, and staff may not have therapeutic backgrounds.
- In homes, caregivers bring their own trauma histories and cultural dynamics.
- In clinics, insurance billing and documentation can create constraints around session length and structure.

Effective scaling begins with listening.

- What's already working?
- Where do staff feel stuck?
- What language will resonate?

DTAP's principles remain the same, but how we teach, coach, and support its delivery must be dynamic.

Protecting Fidelity While Adapting

Scaling a model doesn't mean diluting it. It means adapting it with integrity.

Chaddock protects DTAP fidelity through:
- Clear non-negotiables: The DTAP Pyramid must remain central, with safety prioritized over compliance.
- Certified Ambassadors who understand both the model and the context.
- Fidelity checklists adapted to fit specific settings.
- Regular consultation, reflective supervision, and communities of practice that sustain learning and alignment.

We don't franchise a brand; we nurture a movement. That means prioritizing relationships, ongoing contact, and mutual accountability.

Equipping Leaders as Multipliers

The key to sustainable expansion isn't just training; it's leadership.

When leaders internalize DTAP, they multiply its impact throughout their organizations and systems. That's why Chaddock invests in:
- Executive-level retreats focused on trauma-informed strategic leadership.

- Cross-system collaboratives integrate schools, child welfare, and mental-health leaders to align their approaches.
- Training programs that include mentoring, observations, and community support.

When leaders live the model, fidelity follows.

Advocating for Systems Change

The long-term goal isn't just site-level adoption. It's policy change.

That means influencing:
- Funding models that support relational, non-punitive approaches.
- Training mandates that go beyond "trauma-aware" to trauma-responsive and attachment-based.
- Accountability structures that measure healing outcomes—not just incident reports.

Chaddock engages in state and national advocacy to support this vision.

We share our data. We speak at conferences. We build relationships with policymakers. And we encourage and support other organizations to do the same.

Systemic change requires a shared voice and collective action.

Become a Lighthouse of Hope

Not every organization is ready to fully implement DTAP, but they can still benefit from its guiding light.

We encourage organizations to see themselves as lighthouses: committed to shining the way, sharing what works, and inviting others into the journey.

Scaling isn't about perfection. It's about purpose.

It's about ensuring that more children, in more places, have access to healing relationships.

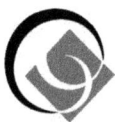

REFLECTION QUESTIONS

As you consider expansion, pause to ask:
- Where does our community need us to shine next?
- Are we expanding for impact, or just for growth?
- How can we remain faithful to the heart of DTAP while meeting the needs of new contexts?
- What systems need to change to make relational healing sustainable and equitable?

DTAP can go wherever people are willing to prioritize healing over control, relationship over routine, and hope over habit.

And the world is waiting.

CHAPTER 8

FAITH AT THE CENTER—SPIRITUAL LEADERSHIP IN A SECULAR WORLD

[This chapter is optional reading for those who want to explore how our faith tradition shapes our leadership—while the Developmental Trauma and Attachment Program [DTAP®] itself remains universally applicable.]

At Chaddock, faith is not an afterthought; it's a foundation. It shapes not only our values but also the way we *are* with one another.

Yet we recognize that in today's diverse and often secular professional environments, talking about faith can feel complicated.

This chapter is about navigating that complexity with grace, clarity, and courage.

Faith as a Guiding Value

We want to be clear: DTAP does *not* require faith to function.

It is a model built on universal principles of healing—Safety, Connection and Regulation, and Reasoning and Competence—that can be applied in any setting, regardless of belief.

But our particular implementation—the Chaddock Way—is deeply informed by our Christian faith.

That faith fuels our commitment to human dignity, the possibility of redemption, and the importance of *servant leadership*. It guides how we lead, how we heal, and how we hope.

The Role of Faith in Healing

Faith creates space for meaning.

Children and families who have experienced profound suffering often seek more than services—they need *hope*.

Faith teaches us to see beyond medical labels and behaviors. It reminds us that healing is not just symptom management but restoration, reconciliation, and belonging.

We've seen children begin to thrive not just because they achieve behavioral stability but because they find purpose and connection.

We've watched staff rediscover their calling in the face of burnout. We've seen families find new beginnings where others saw only endings.

Faith makes room for transformation.

Servant Leadership as a Spiritual Practice

At Chaddock, our leadership model is grounded in servant leadership—a concept rooted in the teachings of Christ, but accessible to anyone who values humility and service.

We believe leaders aren't called to command, but to serve. To listen deeply. To hold people accountable with compassion and truth.

This approach doesn't require every leader to share a specific theology. It simply asks that we lead from humility and service. That we elevate the needs of others and create environments where people feel seen, known, and valued.

Faith-Informed, Not Faith-Imposed

In a diverse workplace, faith should never be weaponized or required.

We offer spiritual reflection, prayer, and Christ-centered mentorship opportunities for those who desire them—but they are always *optional*, never forced.

We are committed to creating a workplace where staff can bring their whole selves to work—including their spiritual identities if they choose.

All individuals are respected and welcomed, whether they identify as Christian, another faith tradition, or no faith at all.

The bond between us is not shared belief but shared dedication to healing through relationships.

Making Space for the Sacred in a Secular World

Many organizations avoid discussing faith out of fear of division.

But we've found that when approached with humility and respect, faith can actually unite.

It reminds us that our work is sacred. That the children we serve carry inherent worth.

That justice, mercy, and love are not just ideals but operational imperatives.

We create space for this through:
- Optional staff devotionals and prayer circles.
- Values-based decision-making guided by shared ethical principles.
- Grief rituals and spiritual care during times of organizational loss.

Faith does not compete with professionalism; it completes it.

It gives heart to our policies and soul to our systems.

Faith in the Face of Burnout

When leaders feel overwhelmed, it's often not strategy they lack; it's spirit.

Faith sustains us when metrics fall short or outcomes come slowly. It reminds us why we started this work in the first place.

As one staff member put it: "It's not just that I work at Chaddock. It's that I'm called to be here."

That's what faith does.

It *calls us*. It *anchors us*. It *renews us*.

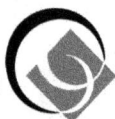

REFLECTION QUESTIONS

As you lead your organization—whether from a place of deep spiritual conviction or quiet openness—consider:

- How are faith, purpose, or meaning shaping your leadership?
- Where do you need renewal, not just professionally, but spiritually?
- How can you lead with both courage and compassion?
- How does your organizational culture make room for hope and dignity without imposing belief?

Faith doesn't require a pulpit.

Sometimes it just requires presence.

And in a hurting world, that presence might be the most healing thing we have to offer.

CHAPTER 9

SYSTEMS CHANGE IN ACTION—LEADING WITH THE DTAP® FRAMEWORK

Trauma-informed care is not just a training or a buzzword.

It's about fundamentally transforming how systems operate so they can truly promote healing, hope, and long-term change.

Many organizations aspire to be "trauma-informed" but stop at surface-level changes—a staff training here, a poster on the wall, a new mission statement.

Real, meaningful change goes deeper.

It challenges us to build systems—organizations, schools, agencies—that live out Safety, Connection and Regulation, and Reasoning and Competence at every stage, for every person.

Chaddock's Developmental Trauma and Attachment Program (DTAP) is not only a clinical approach but a practical, relationship-centered framework for system-wide transformation. Whether you work in residential treatment, schools, community-based agencies, or you're shaping policy at the state or federal level, DTAP offers a road map to create environments where healing truly happens.

This chapter invites you to think beyond interventions to reimagine the very structures, policies, and cultures that shape the daily experiences of children, families, staff—and entire communities.

Why Systems Change Matters

Trauma doesn't just injure individuals.

It shapes entire systems.

Systems built on fear, compliance, or control often recreate the very conditions that retraumatize those they're meant to serve.

Children impacted by trauma arrive with mistrust, dysregulation, and pain. Too often, systems respond with punishment or rigidity. Staff burn out. Families disengage.

Truly trauma-informed systems ask different questions:
- What would it look like to build an organization—or an entire system—where Safety, Connection and Regulation, and Reasoning and Competence aren't just ideas, but daily practice?
- How do we create spaces where staff, families, and children alike feel seen, valued, and supported?

This is not only the responsibility of individual organizations, but of policy leaders who shape funding priorities, regulations, and standards that impact entire systems of care.

Principles of Systems Change with DTAP

The DTAP Pyramid is more than a clinical model. It's an organizational and systems framework to guide culture, policy, leadership, and practice.

Systems change with DTAP is built on these key principles:
- Trauma-Informed Leadership: Leaders model empathy, humility, and curiosity. They create cultures that ask What happened to you? instead of What's wrong with you?
- Integration Across Policies and Procedures: Every policy—from admissions to discipline to staff evaluations—should reflect DTAP principles.
- Staff Support and Well-Being: Caring for caregivers is essential. Trauma-informed systems invest in reflective supervision, relational support, and staff wellness.

- Commitment to Continuous Learning: Systems change is not an event but an ongoing, evolving commitment to growth and improvement.

This work is not just about compliance. It is about living out our deepest values of respect, compassion, and hope—and supporting policies that make such change possible.

Applying the DTAP Pyramid System-Wide

Below, we explore how each part of the DTAP Pyramid can guide change, not only within organizations but across entire systems.

Safety Throughout the System

Safety is the foundation—not just for therapy rooms, but for entire systems of care.

In Residential Care:
- Predictable, calming daily routines
- Intake processes that prioritize trust with families
- Warm, welcoming environments
- Staff training in attunement and co-regulation

In Schools:
- Relationship-based classroom management
- Trauma-informed discipline policies focused on restoration
- Inclusive, culturally responsive learning spaces
- Staff who know and care for students as whole people

In Community-Based Services:
- Transparent, respectful, collaborative intake
- Safe, culturally responsive environments
- Staff who build authentic relationships with the communities they serve

Policy Implications:
- Funding that supports smaller caseloads for relational work
- Regulations requiring trauma-informed and attachment-based training
- Standards that emphasize dignity and family engagement

Connection and Regulation at Every Stage

Connection and regulation are about helping children—and staff—build the capacity to manage emotions, stress, and relationships.

In Residential Care:
- Daily schedules with calming, regulating activities
- Staff trained to recognize and respond to signs of dysregulation
- Response protocols emphasizing co-regulation over control
- Reflective supervision supporting staff well-being

In Schools:
- Teachers trained to recognize student stress

- Calming spaces for students who need breaks
- Predictable routines and transitions
- Staff wellness initiatives to reduce stress and burnout

In Community-Based Services:
- Flexible scheduling to reduce barriers and stress
- Practices validating client emotions with empathy
- Policies supporting time for supervision and reflection

Policy Implications:
- Investing in staff wellness as a quality measure
- Funding reflective supervision
- Standards that prioritize relational over punitive responses

Reasoning and Competence Throughout the System

Reasoning and competence are about building mastery, confidence, and agency for everyone in the system.

In Residential Care:
- Life skills and social skills programming
- Celebrating youth strengths and milestones
- Staff development plans and growth pathways
- Including youth voice in planning and decision-making

In Schools:
- Integrating social-emotional learning into curriculum
- Ongoing professional development for teachers
- Student leadership opportunities

- Staff mentorship and coaching

In Community-Based Services:
- Client-led goal-setting and skill-building
- Staff training and certification pathways
- Celebrating client and staff success stories

Policy Implications:
- Funding for staff development and certification
- Standards supporting client-centered goal planning
- Incentives for cross-sector collaboration to build community competence

Examples of Systems Change in Practice

- **Residential Program Transformation:**
  A facility once reliant on rigid rules transformed its culture using DTAP principles. Staff prioritized attunement and co-regulation. Critical incidents decreased, staff retention improved, and families felt more respected and involved.

- **School Partnership:**
  A district trained all staff in attachment and regulation principles. Discipline shifted to restoring relationships. Teachers created predictable, safe classrooms. Behavior incidents declined and student-teacher trust improved.

- **Community-Based Agency:**
  An agency redesigned its intake process to prioritize trust over paperwork. Staff received training in attachment-focused engagement. Families reported

feeling respected and safe, leading to stronger engagement in services.

Sidebar: Policy and Systems Leadership Implications

Meaningful change depends not just on organizations but on policy leadership at local, state, and federal levels.

Policymakers have the power to:
- Set funding priorities that support relationship-based, trauma-informed care.
- Embed trauma-informed and attachment-based principles in licensing standards, contracts, and grants.
- Invest in workforce development, reflective supervision, and staff wellness.
- Incentivize cross-sector collaboration among child welfare, education, juvenile justice, and mental health systems.
- Support evaluation and accountability that includes Safety, Connection and Regulation, and Reasoning and Competence—not just compliance or behavior.
- Promote equity by removing systemic barriers that disproportionately impact marginalized communities.

Real change happens when policy supports practice.

By championing these principles, policymakers help build systems that not only manage crises but also truly heal.

Practical Steps for Leaders and Policymakers

If you want to lead systems change with DTAP principles:

1. **Assess Your Current Culture:** Where are you strong? Where do you need to grow?

2. **Engage Your Team or Constituents:** Invite honest conversations about change.

3. **Develop a Plan:** Identify clear priorities, champions, and timelines.

4. **Invest in Training and Coaching:** Support staff with knowledge and practice.

5. **Align Policies and Practices:** Revise rules and procedures to match your values and vision.

6. **Commit to Learning:** Build systems for feedback, reflection, and continuous improvement.

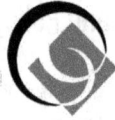

REFLECTION QUESTIONS

As you consider how to apply these steps, pause to reflect on the following questions with your team:

- How do your policies and practices create safety for children, families, and staff?
- How do you support staff in maintaining emotional regulation?
- What opportunities exist to build competence at every stage?
- How can leadership consistently model the values you want to see?
- What is your long-term commitment to this work?

DTAP is not just a clinical model.

It is a leadership framework for building systems that heal by combining the science of healing with the power of relationships.

When organizations and policymakers embed these principles at every stage, they don't just improve services; they transform lives.

And in doing so, they embody the values of respect, compassion, and hope that make true healing possible.

CHAPTER 10

CASE STUDIES AND STORIES FROM THE FIELD

The true power of the Chaddock Way is best understood through the lived experiences of those who have encountered it.

While data, strategy, and structure matter, it's the real-life stories of children, families, and professionals that breathe life into the Developmental Trauma and Attachment Program (DTAP®) framework.

This chapter offers a window into those stories—moments of pain, courage, and transformation that reflect the heart of this work.

Healing in the Cottage: Jasmine's Story

Jasmine arrived at Chaddock's residential program after multiple failed placements. At age twelve, she had already cycled through five different foster homes and two hospitalizations. Her behaviors included chronic running away, explosive aggression, and emotional shut-downs. Traditional behavior management models had labeled her as "noncompliant."

But DTAP asked a different question, not *"What's wrong with her?"* but *"What's happening inside her?"* or *"What's the feeling underneath all of the behavior?"*

Through consistent routines, safe and attuned adults, and predictable expectations, Jasmine began to experience *safety, connection,* and *regulation.* Her direct-care staff practiced co-regulation during meltdowns rather than using punishment. Her therapist helped her identify sensations and label emotions. Slowly, she transitioned from a state of survival to genuine connection.

By her sixth month, Jasmine was building friendships, attending school regularly, and engaging in therapeutic play. Her favorite time was when the staff read bedtime stories—offering her a glimpse of the warmth and comfort she had missed in her early childhood.

She didn't just learn *how* to behave; she learned she mattered.

Transforming a Classroom: Mr. Diaz's Approach

Mr. Diaz teaches fifth grade in a public school that partnered with Chaddock for DTAP-informed classroom training. Initially skeptical, he described his students as "out of control" and himself as "burned out."

After training in regulation strategies and relationship-based discipline, Mr. Diaz shifted his approach.

He began each day with a check-in, asking students how they felt and what they needed. He created a "regulation station" in the classroom—a calming space with weighted blankets, sensory tools, and emotion cards.

The result? Office referrals dropped by 70 percent. Students who once refused to engage became leaders in peer mediation. Mr. Diaz rediscovered his passion for teaching, telling us: "Now I see behavior as communication, not defiance."

Bringing Families Back Together: The Walkers

The Walker family adopted two siblings from foster care, both with histories of neglect and abuse. Despite their deep love and commitment, they struggled with intense tantrums, defiance, and attachment disruptions. Feeling isolated and ashamed, they came to Chaddock for family coaching.

DTAP-based coaching sessions focused on parent attunement, self-regulation, and play-based connection.

Parents learned to identify triggers and co-regulate rather than discipline from frustration. They implemented daily connection rituals: eye contact over breakfast, gratitude sharing at dinner, and ten-minute "special time" with each child.

Six months in, the changes were clear. Meltdowns reduced. Trust grew. One sibling, previously nonverbal during conflict, could now say "I'm scared" instead of acting out.

As Mrs. Walker shared through tears: "DTAP gave us tools, but more than that, it gave us hope."

The Ripple Effect: A Supervisor's Impact

Tonya, a newly promoted residential supervisor, inherited a team with high turnover and low morale. Staff felt unsupported, burned out, and uncertain about how to implement DTAP consistently.

Rather than lead with authority alone, Tonya led with humility and intention.

She introduced reflective supervision meetings and used the DTAP Pyramid as a framework for staff development. She invited her team to identify what helped them feel safe, connected, and competent, just as they would for a child.

Within a year, staff retention improved, incidents of restraint dropped, and team satisfaction soared.

One team member said: "I don't just come to work; I belong to something."

Tonya's leadership showed that DTAP isn't just about clients; it's about culture.

What These Stories Reveal

These accounts represent just a glimpse of the transformative impact DTAP can have when implemented with fidelity, compassion, and courage.

While outcomes vary and the work is never easy, the common thread in every story is relationship:
- Relationship that **sees beyond behavior.**
- Relationship that **prioritizes connection over compliance.**
- Relationship that **builds regulation, competence, and hope.**

In the next chapter, we'll share practical tools to help you lead this transformation in your own organization.

But remember: Every policy, framework, and form must ultimately serve this truth: Healing happens in relationship.

And when those relationships are grounded in Safety, Connection and Regulation, and Reasoning and Competence, transformation is not just possible.

It's inevitable.

CHAPTER 11

THE STRATEGIC PLAYBOOK

Transformation doesn't happen by accident. It happens by design.

Once you've embraced the vision of the Developmental Trauma and Attachment Program (DTAP®) and the Chaddock Way, the question becomes: *How do you lead your team through real, sustainable, strategic change?*

This chapter provides a blueprint for implementing a DTAP-aligned strategic plan, including guidance on how to conduct a two-day planning retreat, engage stakeholders, align culture and systems, and ensure accountability.

Whether you're a CEO, team leader, or external consultant, this playbook equips you with the tools to move your organization from intention to action.

What Makes This Playbook Different

Unlike traditional strategic plans that result in thick binders collecting dust on shelves, the Chaddock approach prioritizes clarity, usability, and alignment.

Your plan should be:
- Simple enough to fit on one to three pages.
- Clear enough for every employee to understand.
- Grounded in real-time organizational culture and capacity.
- Focused on the next three years with actionable, measurable outcomes.

Our goal is to align mission, people, and progress—just as DTAP aligns children's development around Safety, Connection and Regulation, and Reasoning and Competence.

Preparing for the Planning Process

Before the retreat begins, take time for intentional preparation. This phase ensures that your strategic plan builds on honest assessment and shared wisdom.

Recommended pre-work includes:
- Stakeholder Listening Sessions: Include staff, board members, families, and community partners.
- Review of Organizational Data: Financial health, program impact, staffing trends, client outcomes.
- Culture and Values Reflection: Where are you aligned? Where are you drifting?

This work ensures you're not just writing a plan but preparing to lead meaningful change.

The Two-Day Strategic Planning Retreat

Day One: Foundations and Discovery

- Welcome and Framing:
- Begin with a grounding exercise, such as personal reflection on why participants do this work.
- Share the agenda and objectives clearly.
- Vision and Mission Review:
- Are they still clear, compelling, and aligned with your current reality?
- Values Alignment Discussion:
- Invite teams to reflect on where your values show up— and where they don't.
- SOAR Analysis (Strengths, Opportunities, Aspirations, Results):
- Facilitate breakout groups to identify internal strengths and external opportunities.
- Culture Mapping:
- Ask participants to describe the current culture in one word. Then ask: What culture do we want three years from now?
- Team Dinner or Reflection Circle:
- Close Day One with a shared meal or storytelling activity that honors the journey.

Day Two: Focus and Framework

- The Hedgehog Concept Workshop:
- Explore: What are we best at? Most passionate about? What drives our resource engine?
- Three-Year Strategic Framework:
- Define three to five strategic focus areas (e.g., workforce development, service expansion, quality improvement).
- For each area, identify two to three key outcomes and high-level action steps.
- Building Accountability and Ownership:
- Assign champions or leads for each focus area.
- Identify reporting timelines and communication strategies.
- Closing and Commitment:
- Invite each participant to share one commitment they're making to the plan.

After the Retreat—Sustaining Momentum

The work isn't done when the retreat ends; it's just beginning.

Keep momentum going with:
- Regular check-ins on progress.
- Visuals and infographics to simplify the plan for staff.
- Leadership coaching to ensure alignment and support.
- Staff-wide communication and celebration of early wins.

Tools and Templates (Included in the Appendix)

- SOAR Analysis Template
- Strategic Framework Sample
- Focus Area Planning Worksheet
- Strategic Planning Retreat Agenda
- Facilitation Scripts and Prompts

These resources are designed to make the process accessible, practical, and replicable.

Aligning Staff Support with Systems Change

A DTAP-aligned strategy doesn't just address goals and metrics. It requires building a culture where staff feel supported, safe, and valued.

That means:

- Prioritizing reflective supervision and coaching.
- Embedding safety into onboarding, training, and supervision practices.
- Encouraging staff voice in planning and decision-making.
- Investing in wellness, growth, and professional development.
- Building systems that model regulation and competence at every stage of leadership.

Staff support isn't an add-on. It's the strategy.

Grounding the Process in Shared Values

At Chaddock, strategic planning is not just a technical exercise; it's a values-based, relational practice.

We ground every strategic process in reflection and humility, asking questions like:
- *What are we being called to become in this next season?*
- *How do we ensure our plans serve children, families, staff, and our mission?*

We trust that clarity emerges through community discernment and shared insight.

The Strategic Playbook is not just a tool for direction; it's a tool for transformation.

Because when your plan reflects your deepest values, your people come alive, and your mission becomes more than words on paper.

Strategic clarity. Cultural alignment. Missional courage.
That's the power of the Strategic Playbook.

CHAPTER 12

CONCLUSION—BECOMING A LIGHTHOUSE OF HOPE

Every child who walks through your doors carries a story.

Every professional who chooses this field carries a calling.

And every organization brave enough to embrace the Chaddock Way carries the potential to become more than just a service provider.

It can become a lighthouse.

Lighthouses don't remove storms. They don't calm the seas.

But they offer something just as powerful: orientation, visibility, and hope.

They stand firm, grounded in something deeper than the waves crashing around them.

That is what you're building when you implement the Developmental Trauma and Attachment Program (DTAP®) with integrity.

Fostering a Culture of Safety, Connection and Regulation, Reasoning and Competence

You are building a culture rooted in Safety, Connection and Regulation, Reasoning and Competence, where trauma survivors can finally rest.

You are fostering connection so no one has to walk alone.

You are modeling regulation—not only in children, but in staff, teams, and leadership.

You are developing competence, so healing becomes not only possible but sustainable.

And you're nurturing purpose and meaning that anchor your work during the hardest days.

Commitment to Systems Change

DTAP is not simply a clinical model.

It is a leadership framework, a cultural blueprint, and a commitment to systems change.

It invites us to:
- Reflect more deeply.
- Lead more humbly.
- Support staff with empathy and purpose.
- Build systems that don't just manage people but heal them.

Reflection for Leaders

As you close this book, take a moment to ask:
- How will I carry this forward in my work and leadership?
- What conversations do I need to start—or restart—with my team?
- Where is our organization already shining, and where is our light growing dim?

Whether you're starting small or leading system-wide change, remember:
- This is a journey of faithfulness, not perfection.
- Progress will come in inches, not miles.
- There will be hard days.
- But there will also be breakthroughs.
- Moments when a child meets your gaze for the first time.
- When a staff member rediscovers their *why*.
- When a system bends—even slightly—toward healing and justice.

A Call to Shine

You are not alone.

The Chaddock team stands with you.

The DTAP community grows every day.

Most importantly, the children and families you serve are watching—not for perfection, but for presence.

So, stand firm. Stay committed. Shine bright.
Because in a world full of storms, lighthouses matter.
And together, we can light the way.

CHAPTER 13

VOICES OF TRANSFORMATION– TESTIMONIALS FROM THE DTAP® JOURNEY

While research and frameworks matter, nothing is more powerful than the *lived voices* of those transformed through the Developmental Trauma and Attachment Program (DTAP).

The following testimonials come directly from parents, teachers, youth, and professionals who have experienced the Chaddock Way.

From Parents

"For the first time in years, I felt like someone truly saw my child—not just their behaviors, but their pain and potential.

DTAP didn't just help my child regulate; it helped me learn how to be the parent they needed."

—Mother of a nine-year-old

"I used to feel like we were failing as a family. Now we have rhythms of connection and tools to manage tough moments. We're not perfect—but we're closer, calmer, and more hopeful."

—Biological father in Family Coaching Program

From Foster/Adoptive Parents

"Almost two years ago, our son moved in. We were twenty-three and twenty-six and had no idea how to raise an eleven-year-old. All we really knew was that he needed someone who could meet him where he was and show him how special he is.

Through the DTAP program at Chaddock, we received exactly what we needed: support, guidance, and the tools to help him grow. With the help of Chaddock's team and family therapists, he's gone from being reactive and shutting down to staying calm and talking things out.

We've come so far in such a short time. He is calm. He is regulated. He is happy.

Thank you, Chaddock, for making our family whole."

—Foster mom in Foster Care Services

From Teachers

"Implementing DTAP in my classroom changed everything. My students feel safer, and I understand what's happening underneath their behavior. Now I teach not just with my head but with my heart."

—Fifth grade teacher, Public School Partnership

"I used to dread the start of the school day. Now I look forward to our morning circle and seeing the growth in my kids. I finally feel equipped to help, not just manage."

—Special Education teacher

From Youth

"I didn't think anyone would ever believe in me again. But the staff here didn't give up on me. Even when I tried to push them away. That changed me."

—Fifteen-year-old in Chaddock Residential Program

"This place helped me feel like I wasn't broken. They didn't just tell me to calm down; they showed me how to feel safe again."

—Thirteen-year-old outpatient client

From Professionals

"DTAP gave our team a common language, shared values, and renewed energy. We've become more united, more effective, and more committed to healing relationships than ever before."

—Executive Director, Partner Agency

"As a clinician, DTAP shifted my entire treatment lens. It taught me to prioritize Safety and Regulation first—and I've seen clients go further, faster, and deeper because of it."

—Licensed Clinical Social Worker

"It's rare to find a model that's both deeply human and clinically rigorous. DTAP balances both—serving kids with science and with soul."

— Mental Health Consultant, National Training Partner

These stories are not anomalies.

They are the outcome of a model that works, a model that:
- Centers relationships.
- Honors dignity.
- Builds Safety as its foundation.
- Supports Regulation and Competence across every stage.
- Invests in staff well-being and systemic change.

If you're wondering whether DTAP is worth the effort, listen to the people who know it best.

They've lived the change—and they're lighting the way for others to follow.

CHAPTER 14

BRINGING DTAP® TO LIFE—THE PATH TO CERTIFICATION AND FIDELITY

For those inspired by the heart and science of the Developmental Trauma and Attachment Program (DTAP), the next step is clear: transformation through action.

The DTAP Certification Process is the bridge between *inspiration* and *implementation*. It ensures that both individuals and organizations move beyond simply *learning* the model to *living* it daily, with integrity and fidelity.

This chapter offers a road map for understanding and pursuing certification—whether you're a school district, agency, clinician, or leader seeking systemic impact.

Why Certification Matters

Certification isn't just a credential; it's a commitment.

This work requires dedication to uphold fidelity and excellence while maintaining a healing-centered, relationship-based approach.

Certification protects model integrity, ensuring that DTAP implementers deliver services safely, effectively, and consistently, with quality that families and communities can trust.

DTAP is a relational practice that also demands rigorous standards. Certification establishes harmony between core values, essential training methods, supervision, and desired outcomes.

It builds confidence across systems and strengthens trust with families.

DTAP Certification Tracks

Chaddock offers two distinct but interconnected certification pathways:

1. Individual Certification

Designed for therapists, educators, administrators, and other professionals who want to apply DTAP in their own work. Requirements include:
- Completion of DTAP Core Training.
- Successful demonstration of DTAP knowledge and practical application.

- Participation in reflective supervision or consultation.
- Ongoing continuing education in trauma, attachment, and organizational health.

2. Organizational Certification

For agencies, schools, and systems seeking to integrate DTAP principles throughout their entire organization.
Requirements include:
- Full-staff orientation to DTAP (including supporting Safety, Connection and Regulation, Reasoning and Competence).
- Leadership coaching and strategic planning support.
- Development of fidelity monitoring systems.
- Integration into hiring, onboarding, and supervision practices.
- Periodic site review and fidelity assessment by Chaddock.

Certified organizations receive formal recognition as a Certified DTAP Site, along with promotional and consultation support.

Timeline and Commitment

The certification timeline varies based on the size and readiness of the individual or organization, but typical durations are:
- Individual Certification: eight to fourteen months.
- Organizational Certification: twelve to eighteen months.

Certification is renewed every two years to ensure continued fidelity, alignment, and support.

Training Components

DTAP Certification includes comprehensive training in:
- Foundations of Developmental Trauma and Attachment Science.
- The DTAP Pyramid: Safety, Connection and Regulation, and Reasoning and Competence.
- Strategies for co-regulation and repair.
- Trauma-informed supervision and team dynamics.
- Fidelity tools and reflective practices for staff support and quality assurance.
- Strategic planning and leading organizational culture change.

Post-Certification Support

Certified individuals and organizations receive ongoing partnership and resources, including:
- Updated training resources and advanced tools.
- Peer learning communities and annual summits.
- Visibility on the Chaddock website and in promotional materials.

READY TO BEGIN?

If you're ready to begin your certification journey, connect with us:

Chaddock Attachment & Trauma Services
205 South 24th Street, Quincy, IL 62301
Email: **dtap@chaddock.org**
Phone: **217-222-0034**
Website: **www.chaddock.org/dtap**

We believe in your mission.

Let us help you strengthen it—with the power of DTAP.

APPENDIX A

QUICK-START LEADERSHIP ACTION CHECKLIST

Step1: Clarify Leadership Commitment

Gather your executive and board leadership to ensure alignment on why DTAP matters and what transformation will require. This is not just a programmatic shift—it is a cultural commitment.

Step 2: Pursue DTAP® Certification

Contact Chaddock to begin the process of exploring DTAP certification requirements. Early pursuit ensures that your leaders understand the fidelity expectations and can build systems aligned with the model from the outset.

Step 3: Conduct Organizational Readiness Assessment

Assess your organization's current culture, systems, and staff capacity. Identify areas that may need strengthening to fully embrace the transformational change DTAP offers.

Step 4: Facilitate Stakeholder Listening Sessions

Engage staff, clients, and community partners to gather input on strengths, opportunities, and cultural realities. Their feedback will guide strategy and build buy-in for change.

Step 5: Schedule a Strategic Planning Retreat

Design a two-day retreat focused on more than setting goals—its primary purpose is to confirm whether your organization is ready to commit to the cultural transformation that DTAP requires. Chaddock can serve as a resource or facilitator to help guide this process and ensure alignment with DTAP principles. Include cross-functional leaders and key stakeholders in this process.

Step 6: Define Strategic Focus Areas

Using insights from the retreat and listening sessions, identify three to five priority areas for change (e.g., workforce development, practice alignment, culture-building).

Step 7: Establish Accountability Structures

Assign champions for each focus area, set clear metrics, and develop a reporting cadence. Ensure that fidelity monitoring and reflective supervision are embedded from the start.

Step 8: Launch Training and Implementation Plan

Roll out foundational DTAP training for all staff, establish DTAP-Certified Ambassadors or Coaches, and integrate fidelity tools into daily practice.

Step 9: Embed DTAP into Supervision and Hiring

Revise hiring protocols, onboarding, and supervision models to reflect DTAP priorities. Seek staff who value connection, demonstrate resilience, and are open to reflective practice.

Step 10: Celebrate Early Wins and Reinforce Culture

Recognize staff contributions, share success stories, and continuously remind your team why this work matters.

Step 11: Commit to Continuous Learning and Growth

Regularly revisit fidelity data, refine systems, and invest in staff well-being to sustain long-term impact.

Step 12: Tell Your Story

Capture and share your DTAP journey. Your transformation will inspire others and deepen your own organization's commitment to the work.

APPENDIX B

TOOLS AND RESOURCES FOR IMPLEMENTATION

The following tools and resources are designed to help your organization implement DTAP® with fidelity and clarity. Each can be adapted based on the size, scope, and context of your setting.

1. SOAR Analysis Template

Use during strategic retreats or planning sessions to identify:
- **Strengths** – Internal capabilities and values.
- **Opportunities** – External trends and community needs.
- **Aspirations** – Vision for what you hope to become.
- **Results** – Tangible outcomes you want to achieve.

Category	Notes and Reflections
Strengths	
Opportunities	
Aspirations	
Results	

2. Strategic Framework Sample

A three-year plan should focus on 3–5 strategic priorities, each with clear outcomes and leadership.

Strategic Focus Area	Outcome	Lead/Champion	Timeline
Workforce Development	Reduce turnover by 25%	HR Director	Year 1–3
Program Expansion	Launch DTAP in 3 new settings	Clinical VP	Year 2
Quality & Fidelity	Implement fidelity tools system-wide	Program Managers	Year 1–2

3. Focus Area Planning Worksheet

Use to define next steps for each strategic focus area:

- What does success look like?
- What obstacles might we face?
- What supports or resources are needed?
- Who needs to be involved?

4. Strategic Planning Retreat Agenda (Sample)

Day One: Vision, Culture, and Discovery

- Welcome and Team Reflection
- Mission/Vision Alignment Exercise
- Values Mapping
- SOAR Analysis
- Culture Mapping Activity
- Closing Circle or Shared Story Reflection

Day Two: Strategy and Action

- Hedgehog Concept Workshop
- Define Strategic Focus Areas
- Develop Outcomes and Action Steps
- Assign Champions
- Build Accountability Structures
- Final Reflection and Commitments

5. Facilitation Scripts and Prompts

Use these prompts to guide deeper reflection during planning sessions:

- "What does it look like when our mission shows up in our daily work?"
- "Where are we aligned—and where are we drifting?"
- "If a new staff member asked what our culture is like, what would you say?"
- "What's one thing we need to start, stop, and strengthen?"
- "How can we stay true to our values when things get hard?"

6. DTAP Fidelity Observation Checklist

For supervisors, trainers, and coaches to monitor fidelity in action.

DTAP Stage/Domain	Observable Behaviors	Notes
Safety	Environment is calm, predictable; staff use attuned tone, eye contact, presence	
Connection Regulation	Co-regulation strategies actively modeled	
Reasoning Competence	Youth offered opportunities for mastery	

7. Faith Reflection and Integration Tools (Optional)

For faith-based organizations or leaders who want to ground their strategy in spiritual practices.

Note: These are optional and separate from DTAP Pyramid.

- **Scripture for Reflection:** Micah 6:8, Romans 12:2, John 1:14
- **Prayer Prompts:** "What are we being called to release or embrace this season?"
- **Ritual Ideas:** Opening prayer, blessings at milestones, scripture-based affirmations

8. DTAP Certification Readiness Checklist

Assess your organization's preparedness to pursue DTAP Certification:

- Leadership is fully supportive and aligned.
- Staff have completed foundational DTAP training.
- Fidelity tools are in place and regularly reviewed.
- Strategic plan reflects DTAP alignment.
- Ongoing reflection and supervision structures exist.
- Internal trainers are being developed or contracted.

9. Licensing, Certification, and Trademark Use Guidelines

Organizations and individuals must complete and pass the full DTAP Certification process before implementing DTAP in practice.

Certification ensures fidelity to the model, safeguarding its integrity and effectiveness across settings.

To Learn More or Begin the Certification Process:

Chaddock Attachment & Trauma Services
205 South 24th Street, Quincy, IL 62301
Phone: **217-222-0034**
Email: **info@chaddock.org**
Website: **www.chaddock.org/dtap**

We offer:

- DTAP Certification for individuals and organizations.
- Training program pathways.
- Licensing agreements for program integration.
- Ongoing consultation and fidelity monitoring.

Important: Only certified professionals and organizations may present or deliver DTAP-informed services. Certification includes intensive training, practical demonstration, fidelity review, and formal approval from Chaddock. Misuse or misrepresentation of the DTAP framework or name is strictly prohibited and protected under federal trademark laws.

Organizations or professionals wishing to use DTAP must complete the official certification process prior to implementation.

Final Word

The work of healing children and transforming systems is holy ground.

May these tools serve your journey toward clarity, integrity, and relational excellence.

From our team at Chaddock to yours—thank you for shining your light.

APPENDIX C

FREQUENTLY ASKED QUESTIONS ABOUT DTAP®

1. How is DTAP different from other trauma models?
DTAP integrates trauma-informed care with attachment science and organizational leadership. It doesn't stop at behavioral management or awareness—it reshapes culture, relationships, and systems around the core belief that healing happens through safe, attuned, enduring relationships. DTAP guides not just client treatment, but also hiring, supervision, fidelity monitoring, and strategic planning.

2. Is DTAP recognized as an evidence-based or structured model?
Yes. The Developmental Trauma and Attachment Program (DTAP) is listed on the California Evidence-Based Clearinghouse for Child

Welfare (CEBC). This listing recognizes DTAP as a structured, evidence-informed model designed to support children and families impacted by complex trauma and disrupted attachment. Being listed on CEBC affirms DTAP's foundation in established research and best practice while acknowledging its flexibility in diverse real-world settings.

3. Can DTAP be used outside of residential settings?

Absolutely. DTAP was developed at Chaddock's residential campus but is now implemented in outpatient therapy, schools, home-based services, foster care, and coaching models. Its flexibility allows it to serve children and families in their natural environments, while maintaining fidelity to its principles.

4. How long does DTAP certification take?

Certification timelines vary. It will take an individual 8-14 months to complete certification. A typical organization can complete training and certification in 12-18 months. This includes staff training, fidelity tool implementation, and consultation with Chaddock. Individual practitioner certification may be completed in less time depending on training availability.

5. Is DTAP faith-based or secular?

DTAP itself is clinically grounded and evidence-informed, and can be implemented in both secular and faith-based organizations. While Chaddock's organizational culture is shaped by a Christian perspective that emphasizes servant leadership and purpose, DTAP's core principles are universal: Safety, Connection and Regulation, and Reasoning and Competence.

6. How can I get started with DTAP?

Contact us directly to begin your journey.

Chaddock Attachment & Trauma Services

205 South 24th Street, Quincy, IL 62301

Email: **info@chaddock.org**

Phone: **217-222-0034**

Website: **www.chaddock.org/dtap**

REFERENCES

- Collins, J. (2001). *Good to Great*. HarperBusiness.
- Lencioni, P. (2002). *The Five Dysfunctions of a Team*. Jossey-Bass.
- Morford, Kaylee, MA, LCPC. Embracing Resilience: Chaddock's Developmental Trauma & Attachment Program®—Nurturing Attachment Beyond Trauma. Quincy, IL: Chaddock, 2024.

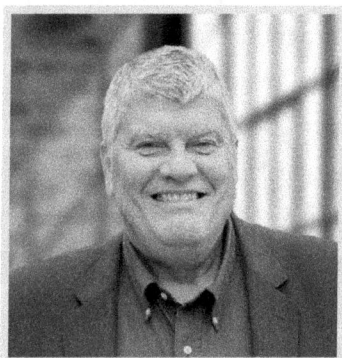

ABOUT THE AUTHOR

Matt Obert, LCSW, is the President and CEO of Chaddock, where he leads a multidisciplinary team dedicated to serving some of the nation's most vulnerable children and families. With over thirty years in the field, Matt has built expertise at the intersection of clinical practice, organizational leadership, and systems change.

Starting as a frontline direct care staff, he has walked alongside youth and families through the hardest moments of their lives, developing a deep commitment to relationship-centered, trauma-informed care. Today, he applies that same relational lens to leadership—working to create organizations that not only talk about healing but live it in every policy, practice, and interaction.

Under Matt's leadership, Chaddock's Developmental Trauma and Attachment Program (DTAP®) has continued to grow to become a nationally recognized framework used by schools, residential programs, outpatient clinics, and policy partners. Matt is a frequent speaker, trainer, and consultant on trauma-responsive leadership, staff well-being, strategic planning, and system transformation. He believes that real change doesn't come from slogans but from courage, humility, and the relentless pursuit of human dignity.

Matt holds a Master's in Social Work and is a Licensed Clinical Social Worker (LCSW). He lives in Illinois with his family and remains committed every day to helping organizations build cultures of safety, connection, and hope.

www.ingramcontent.com/pod-product-compliance
Lightning Source LLC
Chambersburg PA
CBHW070926270326
41927CB00011B/2745